Table of Contents

Quit Sugar! Live Longer! Live Better!

End Sugar Addiction In One Month Or Less and Live A Healthy, Exciting New Lifestyle!

Joe Kozlowski

Introduction

Sugar. Seems harmless enough. However, it is more addictive than cocaine and can lead to numerous health problems such as obesity, diabetes, heart disease, cancer and many other bad things. It can control people the same way narcotics can control people. Sugar is a silent danger, as you don't hear about its effects the same way that you hear about the effects of tobacco and alcohol, but it's a huge danger nonetheless. It's also a manageable danger. One that can be managed so that you can enjoy the sweeter things in life.

The key is to control sugar and not let it control you. Once you end your addiction to sugar, your life will improve in so many ways that you may not have believed was even possible before. You can potentially change your life's path from one full of serious health problems to one with better sleep, more energy, better weight management, and just improved health overall. That's really the goal, to look and feel better overall, right? Otherwise, why quit the sweets?

Thankfully, there's no need to quit them entirely. You can have them (eventually and in moderation) as well as your health. And there are a few ways that you can go about it. Just by making the decision to take action right now, you will put yourself on track to reclaim your life.

It will be difficult in the beginning, but your reward will be a longer, healthier, more fulfilling life. Even if you're feeling sick right now, with some of the health problems mentioned before, quitting sugar could very well be the step needed to slowing down or even reversing those health problems and improving your health. And when you feel healthy, life itself is so much better. And happier.

Ahhhh! A better and happier life. Isn't that worth the
effort? Of course it is! Now let's get started!

Chapter 1

What is sugar and why should I quit it?

Before we start talking about quitting sugar, let's first discuss the basics of sugar. What does it mean when we speak of sugar? Well, there are different types of sugars and some sugars are worse than others. It's always great to know the difference. I'm going to make this short and sweet, no pun intended.

Glucose is the word for sugar that I'm sure you've heard the most. It is the sugar that provides energy to all of the living organisms that inhabit this planet. It is needed by all of the cells and organs in our bodies. Glucose is produced when the food we eat is broken down in our stomachs. From there it is absorbed into our blood stream. Glucose is what is measured in our blood sugar levels. Some sugars are absorbed more quickly, leading to the higher blood sugar levels that wreck havoc on your body. These sugars are the ones that need to be avoided.

Fructose is one of these sugars. Also known as fruit sugar, it is a simple sugar found in many plants. In fact, it is found in honey, tree and vine fruits, flowers, berries, and most root vegetables. It is metabolized differently than glucose and is processed by the liver. Too much fructose can lead to diseases in the liver like non-alcoholic liver disease. It is less likely to be used by the body for energy than glucose and therefore it is more likely to turn into fat. In fact, fructose is more likely to be turned into body fat than fat itself, if you can believe that. And that fat ends up surrounding your liver and other internal organs, which is the unhealthiest place to have fat build up. It's ok to consume fructose in its original form, such as in whole fruit and berries as the fiber and nutrients offset the harm caused by this form of sugar. Even honey is fine in moderate amounts, assuming it's completely natural. However, when fructose, including its baby known as high fructose corn syrup, is added to food during processing, it is almost like poison is added with the potential to do great harm to your health over time. Avoid fructose from processed food as much as you can.

Sucrose is refined white sugar, or the type that you add to your coffee. It is also the type that is added to baked goods. It is the refined, or added, sugar that this book is referring to. It is basically table sugar. Other common names for it is cane sugar and beet sugar. It is composed of both glucose and fructose. It's added to more food products than one can count, generally through food processing. In fact, cutting out processed foods altogether is the best step toward quitting sugar. Refined sugar is found in juices, ketchup, bread, beef jerky, and salad dressings, as well as many other things. Some of those items aren't suspected by most to even have sugar. These foods are processed in such a way that much of the fiber, not to mention many other nutrients, is stripped from them. This loss of fiber is significant as fiber slows down digestion. Without it, the blood stream absorbs sugar more quickly. This raises blood sugar and insulin levels, wrecking havoc on your health. Food manufacturers will try to trick you by calling it cane sugar (which, as stated before is refined sugar by another name), high fructose corn syrup (which is even worse) or some other name unfamiliar to most people. Don't get fooled. Know what you are putting into your body. Other names for refined sugar can be found in **Chapter 8**.

Lactose is a sugar found in dairy that the body can readily convert into glucose (except in those who are lactose intolerant), the main source of energy for your body. It is fine when found in its original form in milk products like natural yogurt and cheeses. It contains many nutrients like calcium and vitamin D. It is composed of glucose and galactose. We've already discussed glucose but let's talk about galactose. Galactose is a healthy sugar that your body needs. It is also known as the "brain sugar" and supports the brain development of babies and children. It is also used as a substance for creating cells in your body. It is even important for your immune system. One thing to note, however, is that many dairy products are processed as well. For instance, the cheap American cheese you find in the supermarket may not even be cheese, but labeled as a cheese product. Cheese products are not necessarily cheese. Just as I have stated before, many times nutritional value is stripped from food during its processing, and that is the case here with cheese products. So **ALWAYS** read the label to know what you are actually consuming!

Sugar can be a lot of different things, as you just found out. Quitting sugar in the end, as is defined in this book, is quitting added or refined sugar, as humans have always consumed sugar in its natural form. However, sugar hasn't become the health problem that it is today until it started being processed into the everyday food that we eat. That is because this added sugar is a substance that our bodies weren't meant to consume. Not to mention that the amounts from the processed food that we eat today in modern times far exceeds the amount of sugar that humans ate before. In fact, according to the American Heart Association, humans aren't supposed to consume more than 7 teaspoons of sugar per day yet Americans consume a daily average of 20 teaspoons. For this reason, I want to stress that quitting added or refined sugar is the real goal here, since that type of sugar is the real danger. Foods containing naturally occurring sugar in its original form, such as in fruits, vegetables and dairy are not driving the sugar related health problems. There may be a few things like honey and agave on which we can overindulge but most of the time the fiber and nutrition that comes from a great array of natural foods in their original form more than offsets any harm that may be caused by their sugar content. And remember, our bodies use it for energy right down to the cellular level. It is the fuel upon which we rely. It's the over-consumption of sugar that is the cause of the diet related illnesses and health problems that we see today.

Avoiding these health problems is worth so much more than the short-term good feeling that you get from sugar as the long-term effects of too much sugar can be downright devastating. And these effects tend to sneak up on people. In fact, some people don't even realize what is happening to them until it is too late. Don't be one of those people. Break this addiction right now. And don't feel bad for having it. Always remember that it's not your fault. As I have said before, the food supply is full of refined sugar and you've been unwittingly consuming it for years, probably since you were a child. It's everywhere. Unless you knew about this already, you would have had a hard time avoiding this addiction. In fact, if you never learned about the prevalence of sugar in everyday food, you'd never break free from its grasp, since you'd never have known you were within its grasp in the first place. Now you have the knowledge to break free. All you have to do is take action and apply that knowledge.

So, what's the cause of sugar addiction? Well, it's the same thing that causes drug addiction. It's the release of dopamine in the reward center of the brain when a large amount of sugar is consumed. This is the same chemical that is released when cocaine and nicotine are consumed. When sugar is eaten often and in large amounts, the dopamine receptors in the brain begin to down-regulate, or reduce, the brain's response to the sugar. This down-regulation leads to fewer receptors for the dopamine. Now more sugar is needed to satisfy the reward center of the brain. This leads to a vicious cycle where more and more sugar is consumed. It's a cycle that can only be broken by changes in habit. Without this change in habit, negative effects eventually occur within the body.

And, wow, what negative effects they are. Aside from that temporary good feeling, refined sugar gives us so little in value. It is full of calories, yet has **NO** nutritional value. **NONE!** That is why the calories that are found in sugar are called "empty calories." There are no proteins, essential fats, minerals or vitamins. All you get is pure energy. Unused, this pure energy unnecessarily taxes the organs and is converted into fat. Consuming too much of the white stuff can also lead to nutrient deficiencies, since calories without nutrients replace others that do have nutrients. Here's another way to look at it Sugar steals nutrition from our diet. And it does so many other bad things as well.

It starts by destroying our teeth. The bacteria in our mouths that cause tooth decay loves that pure energy provided by sugar to give it the energy needed to do what it does best, decay teeth. And tooth decay leads to a poorer diet overall, since it makes it harder to eat real food, which, in general, is harder to chew than processed food, which then leads to, you guessed it, eating more unhealthy processed food. Now we are consuming the dreaded added sugar that we are looking to avoid. Poor dental health is just another way that nutrition can be stolen from our diet by sugar.

The lack of nutrition attributed to sugar also makes it a leading contributor to obesity in both children and adults. However, it's not just those empty calories that cause the obesity but also how our hormones are affected by the sugar. We've already discussed how dopamine levels are affected. There's an important hormone affected as well called leptin. Leptin is the hormone responsible for sending signals to the brain that the body is full. Feeling full is what prevents cravings and keeps calorie intake under control. Too much sugar leads to the body's resistance to leptin. Once the resistance to leptin is developed, the body doesn't feel full after a meal, which leads to more hunger and more sugar cravings. These cravings lead to significantly higher sugar consumption, resulting in sky-rocketing caloric intake, caloric intake that more readily turns into fat if those calories aren't burned. The road to obesity then begins. This is a cycle that people fall into without realizing that they are inside of it. Or at least not until the damage is done. Once a person realizes that he or she is in this cycle, then steps can be taken to break it. In fact, because this cycle is one of the leading causes of obesity, especially in the western world, significantly cutting back on sugar consumption is also one of the best ways to lose weight. If you are overweight, you'll generally notice healthy weight loss once the sugar habit is broken.

And you want to break that habit as soon as you can since excessive sugar is also a major cause of insulin resistance, which is a stepping stone to type II diabetes. Insulin is a hormone that allows blood sugar (glucose) to enter the body's cells from the blood stream where it can be used as energy. It also tells the cells to start burning glucose instead of fat. Too much glucose in the blood stream is highly toxic. This makes insulin very important as it controls how much glucose is in the blood stream, keeping it from spiking. If glucose levels in the blood are consistently higher than they should be, it could lead to the cells becoming "resistant" to insulin, which is needed to control your blood sugar levels. This resistance, if no change in diet and habits are made, will eventually lead to type II diabetes. Type II diabetes occurs when the pancreas can no longer make enough insulin to overcome the body's resistance to insulin. Now there's nothing to prevent the blood sugar levels from getting too high, which leads to heart disease, kidney disease, nerve and blood vessel damage, blindness, foot damage, skin problems, and even cancer. Nobody wants to reach this point, but if you believe that you may have already done so, it's best to consult your physician on which course of action to take next.

And if everything we just went over wasn't bad enough, sugar can even wreck havoc on your sex life. Yes, you read that right! For starters, excessive sugar lowers testosterone. Testosterone is the hormone responsible for sexual health and muscle mass. For men, low testosterone increases body fat. On top of that, excessive sugar also increases estrogen levels, something which can lead to man boobs. These hormone issues can also lead to a low sex drive and erection problems. In women, low testosterone leads to less sexual desire, lower muscle mass, higher body fat and even memory problems. Women who consume too much sugar also tend to have more acne problems, facial hair, and hair loss. Excessive sugar consumption also lowers growth hormones, which is what keeps the body younger. Growth hormones are responsible for maintaining muscle mass, burning and utilizing fat, and keeping up your sex drive. According to researchers, there is a direct link between growth hormones, insulin levels, and sexual function. Too much insulin production, which is caused by too much sugar in the blood stream, reduces your body's ability to produce growth hormones. This reduction in growth hormones then leads to a reduction in testosterone levels, which, as explained before, ultimately leads to a lower sex drive. So are those sweets really worth giving up better and more frequent sex?

After frightening you with all of the negative consequences of too much sugar, let's move on to the positives of removing sugar from your life. There are many terrific reasons, many that you'll notice very quickly.

A big thing one starts to notice is more consistent energy levels and alertness since blood sugar levels are more consistent and stable. Not having those peaks and valleys in energy levels means that there will be fewer periods of time where you will feel tired throughout the day. That mid-afternoon crash experienced by most people will no longer be experienced by you once you have significantly decreased your sugar consumption.

Another reason for those consistent energy levels is the better sleep you'll experience. Excessive sugar can cause sleep disruption. People who significantly reduce their sugar intake tend to notice better sleep and can even experience relief from insomnia. On top of that, when you are able to sleep better, you are less prone to the hunger hormones that increase due to poor quality of sleep, preventing cravings and making it easier to continue your new sugar-free lifestyle.

You will then be more inclined to make healthier food choices. As in healthier food with little to no added sugar. And when you cut out or significantly reduce the refined sugar from the food that you eat, then the food you eat will more likely have the nutritional essentials such as vitamins, minerals, fiber, protein, healthy fats, as well as other good stuff. In fact, foods without refined sugar, you will find, tend to be very healthy. Many are also very tasty. You will start changing your diet to include these healthy, tasty foods, which will become part of your lifestyle. This will lead to several other positive changes in your health.

One of those changes involves your weight. When people fail with their diets, the biggest reason for their failure is their inability to handle the sugar cravings. Having said that, if losing weight is your main goal, managing those sugar cravings should be your first step. And when you are able to maintain a lifestyle where sugary foods are replaced by healthy alternatives, not only do you get the essentials your body needs to stay healthy while satisfying your hunger, but you also maintain higher energy levels, as mentioned earlier. You may even have some energy left over for exercise, which will help you lose the weight even faster, not to mention help you boost your energy and improve your health so much more quickly than just changing your diet alone. Are you starting to see how one or two changes can domino into life changing results?

On top of losing weight, reducing sugar consumption also reduces inflammation in the body. This is quite important since inflammation can cause the systems in our body to slow down and not function properly, which includes the immune system, leading to more illness. In fact, inflammation is the root cause for most disease and many times the root cause for chronic, ordinary pains, such as back or foot pain. So if you cut out the sugar you can cut out the sick days (at least the ones where you're really sick). You'll also cut out the nagging little pains that affect many of us on a regular basis.

Sick days and nagging little pains aren't the only things that we want to stop. We also want to stop feeding the cancer cells, as refined sugar does just that by providing these cells with the energy needed to destroy other cells. By reducing the amount of sugar consumed, there is a greater chance of preventing many types of cancer. Reducing sugar also aids in preventing the replication of malignant cancer cells throughout the body. Cancer is no joke. I'm sure you'll agree that it's worth preventing.

Avoiding the sweet stuff also allows you to protect the liver. Excessive sugar can lead to a toxic build-up in the liver, similar to what occurs when one consumes too much alcohol. Reducing sugar consumption, especially consumption of fructose, will lead to reducing that toxic build-up.

Your heart will thank you too. Excessive sugar is linked to lower HDL, or good cholesterol. Reducing it can lead to increasing your HDL (good) and reducing your LDL (bad). It can even help you ditch cholesterol medications once your cholesterol levels are within the normal range. This is a good thing since cholesterol medications can tax internal organs like the liver.

There are just so many areas in your life that can be

significantly improved simply by reducing your sugar intake. Don't you want to claim a better and healthier life? If you do, which I'm sure is the case if you've read up to this point, then continue on to the next chapter and see what you can do to quit sugar right now.

Chapter 2

What can I do to quit sugar?

Before you start executing any plan to quit sugar, you need to get into the right mindset. Your mindset will have more to do with whether you succeed or fail than anything else. Without the proper change in how you think, you will not be able to take the action that you need to take and do it consistently. Failure and frustration is then sure to follow.

As with anything, to be successful you have to set yourself up for success. When it comes to quitting sugar, don't just leave sugary foods in your kitchen and tell yourself that you are not going to eat them, unless, that is, you want to set yourself up for failure. Throw it all out or give it away. If you know that the sugary food is there, you are more likely to crumble and have a "little" something. That "little" something can turn into a "big" failure. I am quite sure that is not what you want. Instead, fill up your cupboard with protein laden foods, foods with healthy fats and foods with fiber. Filling your cupboard with healthy food will give you great choices for satisfying your hunger while still avoiding sugar. Success will then be so much easier.

And while you are setting yourself up for that success, stop looking for loopholes when it comes to your diet. Always keep in mind that refined sugar is not food. It's a poison that slowly kills you. For instance, you may have heard things like, "eat something sugary that you crave, and then eat something healthy right after it" or "eat sugary food slowly and savor it" or other things like it. There's only one problem. You're still consuming sugar instead of breaking away from it. It's still controlling you. If you're looking to break the addiction, then you need to understand that any sugar can sabotage your success in the beginning. Even fruit can be a problem (depending on the level of your sugar addiction) when you are in the initial cold turkey stage since it generally has some sugar. As long as you continue the struggle and not give in to the excuses, you will be doing better than most people.

In fact, most people won't even try to stop eating sugar even after learning about the problems that it causes. Don't be like most people. Many times success happens for people because those people do the opposite of what most everyone else is doing. Following the herd can lead you to slaughter. Sometimes even off a cliff. Or in the case of sugar, bad health.

Now if you want to take action, there is one warning I want to give. One mistake that most people who take action do is to try to do too many things at one time. That is another road to frustration and possibly failure. You should do the opposite. When it comes to quitting sugar, until you have it beaten, stick to focusing just on that. Don't add weight loss, becoming a vegan, or some other major life change to your plate. Besides, quitting sugar can be a great initial step for one of those goals. Once you have sugar licked, then move on to something else.

Support is also key to your success. Quitting with a buddy and holding each other accountable will give you more will power to continue the process and therefore, a greater chance at success. Supportive people strengthen your resolve, pushing you to be more successful. However, you need to be mindful of telling the wrong people. Doing so can increase the chance for failure, or at least make the process to your ultimate success a little more painful. Some people may try to sabotage you because they are jealous that you are improving yourself while they aren't getting anywhere. Some people just don't believe eating sugar is even an issue in general and may think that you are crazy for putting yourself through such a process. These types of people are more prone to ask you to try some sugar-filled food, saying things like, "A little bit won't hurt" or "You can eat a little less tomorrow." They may even guilt you into breaking your new lifestyle by saying, "But I made it myself!" Now, remember, not everyone is trying to keep you from bettering yourself, it's just a lack of understanding on the part of some people. That doesn't make the consequences of giving in to them any less harmful. You just have to be firm when you decline their generous offer. Oh yeah, and always be polite, at least at the start. You don't want to lose friends unnecessarily. Another point, always ignore people who are just negative. In fact, avoid them if at all possible. They never have anything to add that will help you in any way.

A proper mindset also includes an understanding that the small decisions count. Here's what I mean. It is true that having one can of soda today isn't going to negatively impact your health in the long run. It is also true that if you have water in place of that soda today that it is not going to positively impact your health in the long run either. However, if you have that thought every day, over the long term, you will have that soda every day in place of that glass of water and become unhealthier overall for it. Choose the water single every day and it will lead to great health benefits over the long run. So start now! Don't fall into that trap!

Always look at the big picture during the process of quitting sugar. Always keep it in your mind. Breaking sugar addiction is a long-term goal that never ends. You will always need to think about that every single time that you make a decision about what to eat, but in the end, all the benefits, including better health, feeling more energetic with less pain and just an overall better quality of life will make everything well worth it.

There are some tricks that you can use that will help you break the hold that sugar has, which is stronger than most people realize. These tricks are a great place to start as figuring out where to begin when quitting sugar can be very overwhelming.

The first thing that you need to do is to learn how to read nutrition labels. If you just start walking around the grocery store and look at the labels, you'd be amazed at the types of foods where sugar is found as well as the amount of sugar processed into those foods. Food manufacturers add sugar to these foods to make them taste better so they can sell more with little regard for public health. The government doesn't really do anything about it either. That's why you have to take responsibility for yourself and study the labels. Sugar can be found in foods such as ketchup, spaghetti sauce, salad dressings, dried fruit and many other things. It's refined sugar that does the most harm to your health, since it is added during the processing of these foods while the nutrients are stripped away. And it generally makes up the majority of most people's diets. In fact, this food processing is how sugar addiction was imposed on us at a very young age. And there was very little chance of understanding what we were doing to our bodies. Why? Because it was introduced by our parents and others who also didn't know what was in the food they gave us, underestimating the dangers posed by sugar. That's why this isn't the same as drug addiction, where in

most cases, the user made an active choice. Even though
sugar is like a narcotic, neither you nor the people who fed
you while you were young knew its risk for addiction.
That's because there is so much food around containing
significant amounts of sugar that most people don't even
suspect to have sugar. But now you know that sugar can be
anywhere. All you have to do to find it is to read the label.

Looking at the label is not enough, however. You also need
to know how to find sugar on the label and when it comes
to sugar, it is known by many different names. You pretty
much want to read the label of any processed food because,
as I have said before, refined sugar can be found in the
most unexpected places. Here are some of its names as
given by the U.S. Department of Health and Human
Services: *anhydrous dextrose, brown sugar, cane crystals,
cane sugar, corn sweetener, corn syrup, corn syrup solids,
crystal dextrose, evaporated cane juice, fructose sweetener,*
and *fruit juice*. There are other names as well. You don't
really need to know the differences between these terms but
at least be familiar with them. Just identify them as refined
sugar when you see them on the label. In fact, just assume
that any ingredient that ends in **-ose** is another word for
sugar. There's additional information about the different
names of refined sugar in **Chapter 8**.

While reading the label, also note that the ingredients are
listed in descending order according to their weight. In
other words, the ingredient that makes up the most weight
in a food product will be listed first. So if an ingredient
that you know as another name for sugar is listed at or near
the beginning of the list of ingredients, assume that it has a
large amount of sugar. Also note that anything that should
have fat but is labeled as no fat, low fat, or reduced fat will

almost certainly have added sugar in it. And definitely more than its standard version. You also want to avoid artificial sweeteners, which may not be sugar, but they can still increase sugar cravings when ingested. In fact, avoid anything that is marketed as "sugar-free" as it will have those very sweeteners that you want to avoid.

Also cut out sugary drinks as doing so will take you a long way towards your goal. Most drinks have sugar added to them, with the obvious ones being fruit juices and soda. However, you'll find it in specialty coffee and iced tea as well. The problem with sugar from drinks is that all of that sugar enters the bloodstream quickly since there's no fiber (like in fruit) that will slow down the digestion of the sugar and ultimately slow down its absorption into your bloodstream. This will cause blood sugar levels to quickly spike. Eventually your blood sugar levels will then crash leaving you tired and craving more sugar. These types of drinks also increase cravings due to the fact that your appetite isn't being satisfied by their consumption. This means that you'll still be hungry. The best way to avoid sugar when thirsty is to just drink water. Drink water even when you're hungry, as we tend to confuse thirst with hunger nowadays. Doing so will lead to less caloric intake. Water also has many health benefits. It increases energy, flushes toxins (including sugar), promotes weight loss, improves complexion of the skin, boosts the immune system and so much more. You don't get any of this from even the healthiest of fruit juices. Well, maybe you get fatter. Wrapped up in one sentence, eat your calories, don't drink your calories.

When you eat your calories, however, make sure that they don't come from simple carb sweet treats. These include, but are not limited to pastries, cookies, muffins, and any other foods that are made from refined flour. These treats not only lack nutrition but are full of refined sugar. You want to replace these carbs with the type of carbs that you receive from whole grains. Whole grains are full of fiber. Examples of whole grains include whole wheat, oats, brown rice, barley, corn, quinoa, rye, buckwheat, and millet.

Fiber is so essential to help wean you off sugar. It helps to satisfy your appetite, which stops the cravings and keeps your blood sugar levels stable. When substituting sugary processed foods (which, again, is stripped of fiber as well as other nutrients) with fruit, for example, the fiber allows for slower digestion, which then allows the sugar in the fruit to be released into the blood stream more slowly, instead of the rush from something like cake or candy. Fruit also has nutrients. The sugar in fruit is more than offset by its fiber and its nutrients. It is a great replacement for sweets. Some say it's best not to even eat fruit in the first two weeks of quitting. That's a personal choice. Not eating fruit during the initial quitting period can end the addiction more quickly but can also make the quitting process more difficult. Of course, vegetables are a great source of fiber too. Don't just stop with fiber, however.

Add fat to the diet as well. Fat has been demonized in our culture for decades and this demonization has lead to fat being replaced by refined sugar in the American diet. If you haven't noticed, obesity has significantly increased in the United States since this cultural dietary shift from a high-fat low-sugar diet to a low-fat high-sugar diet. And obesity brings its own set of health problems of which I'm sure you are aware. Now when I say eat more fat, I don't mean fried fats or trans fats, but healthy fats which are the unsaturated fats. Unsaturated fats include polyunsaturated fats and monounsaturated fats. Healthy fats are also a source of energy that can replace sugar. Have them with every meal. They will leave you feeling fuller so you will feel less hungry with fewer cravings while maintaining more consistent energy levels. Examples of foods with healthy fats include avocados, seeds, nuts, and fish with omega 3 fatty acids. Another way of adding healthy fats to your diet is to cook with olive oil or to pour a little bit on some cooked vegetables or on a piece of whole grain bread.

Protein is also essential with every meal. There are animal based proteins and plant based proteins. Some sources of animal based proteins are chicken, pork, eggs, and fish. Plant based proteins come from sources such as quinoa, buckwheat, tempeh, hemp, and chia seeds. Always try to eat protein with every meal if you can as it helps keep you feeling fuller longer.

I can't stress enough how important it is to prepare your food from scratch, as you will have better control into what is in your food and, therefore, what is going into your body. We'll discuss later what foods to eat and what foods to avoid in more detail. However, to keep things simple, do your grocery shopping in the produce, meat, and dairy sections of the supermarket. The processed foods from the middle section of the supermarket is where all of the added, or refined, sugar is found. Failure can be found there as well.

Supplements can be a useful tool to help you with balancing out blood sugar levels. Chromium is a mineral needed for balancing blood sugar levels and there's evidence that adding it as a supplement can reduce sugar cravings. Taking B complex vitamin supplements can help with cravings as well. Probiotic supplements are something else to consider since it purges yeast from your system. Yeast feeds off of sugar so ridding your body of said yeast will decrease the cravings too. Adding a good fiber supplement can help if you don't have great access to fresh vegetables and whole grains, although the best option is to get fiber from your actual meals. Adding a few tablespoons of chia and sprouted flax into your diet can also help to add fiber in a pinch.

Exercise can have a major effect on your cravings. In fact, moderate exercise releases the same hormones as chocolate, which helps you feel good and also helps with balancing blood sugar levels. Not to mention, it will help you in losing the weight gained from your sugar addiction. You are also less likely to be bored. Many times we eat for stimulation and sugary foods are where many of us turn for that stimulation. The type of exercises you choose can make a difference in managing your cravings. Excessive cardio, for example, can increase them. Weight training and isometric exercises, such as yoga, however, help stabilize blood sugar levels so that you won't crave carbs and sugars, which is ideal for reaching your goal. So reduce the long distance cardio workouts, like jogging. If you want to continue to do cardio, then do interval training, which more resembles weight training in terms of how it stabilizes blood sugar levels. Run/walk and sprint/jog are examples of interval training. In other words, run hard then walk during the rest period and repeat. An example is to run for three minutes, walk for one minute, then keep repeating it. You can make the intervals whatever you like but make sure that you are challenging yourself or it will be more like straight cardio. Once you get in better shape, try sprinting 100 yards, then walking 100 yards and repeat. Start with ten times and keep increasing. Always keep challenging yourself. Your body will feel stronger in the long run.

Not only does it make you stronger, but exercise also helps manage stress, which is another key to ending sugar addiction. The way stress is managed can very much impact cravings. High stress raises cortisol levels, which causes hunger and increases sugar cravings. So don't let the little things get to you. If there are things or people that cause stress in your life, avoid them if at all possible. Also get plenty of sleep (eight hours is preferred) as being well rested helps lower stress levels. Sleep is also important because poor sleep increases the release of hunger hormones. These hormones can lead to bad decision making in your diet as you look to get that quick boost in energy levels that sugar provides, until the inevitable crash, that is. Then those cravings return, beginning a vicious cycle of bad decisions. Do what you can to avoid stress triggers, including getting plenty of good sleep.

Here are some other random things to try. After a meal, brush your teeth right away as you are much less likely to want to eat any sugary foods when there is that minty taste in your mouth. Also keep healthy snack options within easy reach. These include, but are not limited to, full fat and Greek yogurt, nuts, seeds, and vegetables with a dip like hummus and guacamole. Introducing sour foods into your diet is a great option as well. It helps with reducing the desire for sweet tastes. Try a lemon or lime in your water or a grapefruit as a snack. Keep in mind that sour tastes may take getting used to while your taste buds are retrained.

Portions are another thing to keep in mind. Always understand exactly what makes up one serving. Many things that you eat will seem like one serving, but if you check the label, you may find two servings or more. So the five grams of sugar you thought you were consuming may actually be ten or fifteen grams. This is yet another reason to religiously read the labels. Measure everything out if you have to. For example, if your favorite cereal has a serving size of one cup, then measure out exactly one cup of that cereal. See exactly how much cereal that is. You may find that the bowl you eat every morning is three cups, or three servings, not one. Understand what you are consuming at **ALL** times! A lack of understanding will lead to a lack of results.

Another thing worth trying is to simply chew your food longer. Not only are you able to spend more time savoring your meal, but you also give your body a chance to feel satisfied so you are less likely to feel hungry when you've finished that meal. This leads to less calorie consumption and ultimately less sugar consumption. Chewing your food longer is worth the time and is underrated as a way to minimize overeating. It also helps your stomach digest the food more efficiently.

Reducing sugar consumption is **NOT** a temporary diet change but a new lifestyle. It will be a new lifestyle full of possibilities and greater health. You will still need to learn how to wean yourself off sugar. Check out how in the next chapter!

Chapter 3

How should I quit sugar? Cold turkey or gradually?

What steps should I take to quit sugar? Should I go cold turkey with complete detox (at the start) or gradually wean myself off sugar? Those are common questions for people with a strong sweet tooth that they're looking to ditch. There's no easy answer. Remember, just making the decision to change will get you further than deciding to do nothing. One will get you there faster. The other will just make you take more time to get there. However, not doing anything will get you nowhere.

The best and fastest way to wean off sugar is to quit it cold turkey. Before you can go cold turkey, however, you must first identify which foods and drinks contain sugar. This requires reading and understanding the food labels. When looking at the labels, you need to look for the word "sugar" as well as words that are more or less synonyms for sugar. Remember that words ending in **-ose** are essentially sugar by another name. You have to look at the labels of everything in your diet as sugar is not only found in sweets like candy and bakery items but also in things that you may not even suspect such as sauces, bread and even pizza. So, I repeat, read the labels as the more knowledge you have about the enemy, the better your strategy can be to defeat the enemy. And treat sugar like your enemy as it is a substance that threatens your health and anything that threatens you should be treated as such.

Once you've taken stock of what is in your diet sugar-wise, get rid of the items that contain sugar. Throw them away or give them away. It doesn't matter. Then find a date to start going cold turkey. It's best to start right away, as many of us say that we'll do something tomorrow and we all know how that usually goes. Having said that, some of us may need time to mentally prepare for the challenge of going cold turkey on sugar. Do what is best for you as the only important thing is that you follow through. Try to mentally approach this challenge by reminding yourself of the positive benefits you'll reap such as breaking the addiction, losing weight, and becoming healthier in general. Purge from your mind how much you'll miss your favorite sugary snack or the awful withdrawals. That's the addiction talking. Cocaine and heroin addiction say the same thing. Always look past the darkness to see the joyous light at the end of the tunnel.

Once you start going cold turkey, you will want to avoid, at a minimum, all of the foods that include refined, added sugar as well as the foods that easily convert to sugar, such as those containing refined grains and flour. Examples include white bread, bagels, breakfast cereals, candy, etc. There is more information on these foods in **Chapter 5**. Instead, eat foods with plenty of fiber, protein, and healthy fats. Examples of these include fresh fruits, vegetables, nuts, lean meats like chicken breast and salmon, as well as other nutrient dense foods. There is more information on them in **Chapter 6**.

After a short time of going cold turkey, you will notice withdrawal symptoms, or side effects. Many people, after a few days, experience more cravings, low energy levels, irritability, headaches and dizziness. This is normal as your body is adapting to the new sugar-free diet. In other words, your body is adapting to the new normal that you are setting for it. It's another thing for which you must be mentally prepared. Again, think of the benefits as you fight your way though these challenges. Also drink plenty of water and eat plenty of vegetables, fruits, nuts and other healthy foods to kill the hunger and help alleviate these side

effects. You will know that you have weaned yourself off
of sugar once your cravings disappear and your energy
levels stay consistently high.

How long does it take to be weaned off sugar cold turkey?
It depends who you ask. You may find answers stating
anywhere from a week to a month. I would say two weeks
is the amount of time it takes for the cold turkey process to
work as your taste buds need to adjust as well as your body.
Once your body and taste buds have adjusted, I would be
very careful about reintroducing sweets as well as refined
flours and grains. This may lead you back to the same road
of addiction that you were on before. If you decide to have
a cookie, make sure that your discipline is in place to stick
to just one or before you know it you've eaten an entire
package. If you don't trust yourself to have just one, do
yourself a favor and just say no, as Nancy Reagan would
say. Everything you've worked so hard for is so much more
important than what you can get from one treat. Ending an
addiction with a substance like sugar is a major
accomplishment. Don't throw that away!

I do understand that going cold turkey is a hard, difficult
way to wean yourself off of sugar. However, it is not the
only way. It can most definitely be done gradually.
Sometimes, when it comes to making major changes, and
quitting sugar is definitely a major change, it's best to try to
keep things as simple as possible and not make the changes
too drastic. And there's a good reason for this. Most
people, myself included, lack the discipline to just change
their entire lifestyle on a dime. And that's OK too. Just
start with small changes. For instance, you can start by
replacing the sugary drinks you currently consume with
water. Or you can just as easily replace the morning donut

with an orange. Just make one change first. Once you can handle the first change, then make another. And when you can handle that change, make another one. Just keep making those small positive changes. They will lead to big steps on the road to better health. Eventually, everything will change. And for the better too.

Understand that some people can change more quickly than others. If you can make more drastic changes and stick with them, then go ahead and do it. Keep in mind that if you have a moment where you fail, like binge eating candy or cake, or having five cans of soda at a picnic, it's OK. Let me repeat, it's OK. Nobody is perfect. I'm sure you knew that already but sometimes we as human beings just need to be reminded of that very fact. Just go back to the positive changes that you made before and forget that the weak moment you had ever existed. Don't ever let one bad occurrence or even one bad day get you down. Not even a bad week or a bad month. If you fall down, just get back up again and keep going.

The one advantage that you have from gradually weaning yourself off sugar is that you won't be hit as hard by withdrawal symptoms in comparison to going cold turkey. And for that reason, for many people, the new sugar-free lifestyle will have a better chance to stick since the cravings will be less intense. It also allows you to more easily introduce it into your life instead of causing an upheaval in it. However, you won't get to that sugar-free lifestyle as quickly as you would by going cold turkey. Maybe it's better if you just start gradually. Just learn what you like to eat without sugar, become better at reading and understanding the labels and then go cold turkey. Going cold turkey is more painless when you are better educated on your sugar-free options.

Just don't get too hung up on whether it's better to go cold turkey or to wean yourself gradually as it's really only about replacing those empty calories from sugar with nutritious calories from fiber, protein, and healthy fats. Consume calories that provide your body with what it needs instead of calories that provide it with nothing. That, above all, will lead you to that healthy lifestyle being sugar-free effectively brings. The most important thing, and I can't emphasize this enough, isn't whether to wean sugar out of your diet or to go cold turkey, but to make the decision to become healthier by ending your sugar dependence. And then to take action on that decision. Without taking proper action today, tomorrow won't be any better than yesterday. And that is such a sad thing. I know you'll make it happen. I know that tomorrow will be better.

Chapter 4

What should I prepare for when I quit sugar?

There are a whole lot of things that happen when you drastically lower your sugar consumption. Obviously many of those things are good or why bother? And the good will far outweigh the bad while also lasting longer. In other words, your quality of life will drastically improve in exchange for some short term pain. That short term pain is just the symptoms from sugar withdrawal. Let's go through what that is, as mental preparation will lead to a greater chance of success.

It will be a difficult process initially when you drastically cut your added sugar intake. As I stated in the previous chapter, if you slowly replace sugary foods with healthy replacements, the symptoms will be far less intense than going cold turkey, but the results won't come as quickly. Either way, you will have to push through these symptoms in order to forever change your life for the better. The length of time you've been addicted to sugar and the amount of sugar consumed during that addiction period will also determine the intensity of the withdrawals. These withdrawal symptoms are something for which you need to be prepared. Let's go through many of the things that you will go through.

One of those things is anxiety. Sugar, at least in the short term, makes us happy, specifically because of the released dopamine. When it's taken away, our brains can't help but react. It may give you some jitters, even causing you to have shaky hands at times. Taking away sugar can even lead to depression. And because these things are caused by your body receiving less sugar than it's used to, your cravings will become more intense than ever before. These cravings will need to be fought with the heart of a champion as giving into them will bring you back to square one. Defeating the cravings will end sugar's control over you once and for all and allow you to enjoy a healthier, more fulfilling life.

These cravings are generally accompanied by hunger. Satisfy that hunger with nutrient dense foods that contain protein, fiber, and healthy fats. Examples of those foods can be found in **Chapter 6**. Natural sweeteners like cinnamon can also help. Like I said in the previous chapter, chromium B complex vitamin and probiotic supplements are usually helpful with cravings. Even a piece of whole fruit can help, as added sugar is the real enemy, although I would limit fruit to just one or two servings per day during the first couple weeks after quitting. Some may say to eliminate it altogether. If you just want to greatly reduce sugar consumption, you probably don't need to get so drastic as to eliminate fruit entirely.

Impulsiveness is something that is also commonly experienced. In fact, it's experienced by people quitting addictions in general, including drugs and alcohol. It may lead you to transfer your sugar addiction to other areas of your life. This may include increased smoking, drinking, gambling, shopping and other activities which can negatively impact your life and your health. Try doing more activities that are healthier or more productive like biking, yoga, tai chi, reading, and the like. Anything that takes your mind off of sugar without hurting you somewhere else. This can help reduce the crankiness you may experience in this process as even the calmest and most rational people can struggle with controlling their emotions and behaviors while kicking addictions, sugar included. If you have to be addicted to something, then make it something that adds to your life and experience, not take away from it. Just be aware that you may go through some irritability, which is nothing to be surprised about and is completely normal.

Low energy will also have you down a bit. You may feel the need for more naps and if you take them, find that they can last significantly longer. There's a reason for this. When your body has been conditioned to use sugar as its go-to source for energy, it will become lethargic when that source is significantly reduced or stopped altogether. When you change your diet to have more (healthy) fat and protein, it will take time for your body to adjust. Once it does, it will be able to efficiently receive energy from those sources. The result of this being that you will no longer experience the boom and bust energy cycles from the high sugar diet, but instead have a more consistent energy level with less feeling of tiredness throughout the day.

Strong headaches are another symptom that can occur. In fact, they are quite common. A small amount of sugar can help. Get that sugar from fruit such as watermelon, apples, and blueberries. Keep hydrated with water as well. Obviously, stay away from junk food. If the headaches become too much to bear, try quitting more gradually. There's nothing wrong with slowing down. Just understand that if you're moving in the right direction that you'll reach your destination eventually.

Here are some other symptoms that you may experience:

- Insomnia
- Weird Dreams
- Nausea

- Chills
- Sweats
- Muscle Aches and Pains
- Constipation or Diarrhea
- Strong Hunger
- Overeating/Possible Weight Gain
- Strong Thirst
- Frequent Urination

Remember that you won't experience all of these symptoms but you'll experience at least a few of them with varying degrees of intensity. It will be difficult, but always remember that the difficult times will end. You can bet on that.

And when those difficult times do end, you will find yourself feeling better and looking better with overall better health. Many health conditions can even start to reverse themselves after a period of time. This includes, but is nowhere near limited to, diabetes, obesity, and high cholesterol. That in and of itself makes staying the course not only worthwhile, but possibly one of the best decisions of your life. What can be better?

Chapter 5

What common foods should I avoid?

(Or at least limit)

Quitting sugar does mean one thing. And that one thing is to stop eating and drinking some of the things that you just absolutely love. Or at least to limit their consumption. However, don't fear, as there are definitely some tasty replacements. Keep in mind that once you start reaping the health benefits from quitting or significantly reducing your added sugar intake, this will not seem like a such a sacrifice at all. It's always difficult in the beginning but finding replacements for the foods on this list is easier than you might think. Now here are the foods that you will need to ban (or at least significantly limit) from this moment going forward:

Candy

There's a lot that could be said, but does it really need to be? Just avoid it altogether. There is nothing beneficial that your body receives from candy. And don't keep it stashed anywhere. If you do have any, just give it away or throw it away.   It's hard not to eat it when you know you have it stashed. It's so much better to stash healthy snacks instead like fruits or vegetables.

Sugary Drinks

I know this was already explained earlier but it's so important that it is worth mentioning again. Sugary drinks are very bad, as they spike your blood sugar levels very quickly as there is nothing in the way of fiber to slow their digestion. The excess sugar in your blood then gets stored as fat in the liver, which is the most dangerous place for fat to be stored in the body. These drinks are probably the biggest drivers in the rise of obesity and diabetes simply because liquids don't satisfy an appetite like food does, allowing people to consume a ton more sugar and calories than they otherwise would with solid food. Sugary drinks include, but are not limited to, soda, fruit juices, iced tea, and energy drinks. In fact, most drinks that are not water will probably have sugar. The best advice to follow is to just drink water when thirsty, which is one of the healthiest things that you can do anyway. Drinking water will also save you money as it costs much less than those sugary drinks (many times free), leaving you with more money to spend on healthier food. If you want to add a little flavor, just add a slice of lemon.

Dried Fruit

Dried fruit sounds healthy. And I suppose it's better than candy. However, when fruit is dried, the sugar becomes more concentrated. For example, if you take a half cup of fresh cranberries, you get two grams of sugar. A half cup of dried cranberries, on the other hand, has 37 grams of sugar. See the difference? Raisins are also included in this category. Always keep in mind that when the water content is taken out of fruit, the fruit becomes less filling, leading to the possibility that even more dried fruit, and ultimately much more sugar, is eaten. Dried fruit also has preservatives which isn't healthy to consume either. Always eat whole fruit whenever you want to eat fruit.

Bottled Salad Dressings

Anybody who decides to eat a salad is making a conscious decision to eat healthy. Little would that person know that once he or she adds any one of the many salad dressings found at the local grocery store that the salad itself is sabotaged. Why is this? Well, because many salad dressings are manufactured with sugar and high fructose corn syrup. Especially the fat-free and reduced-fat ones. Instead of adding sugar to your salad by putting dressing on it, you can instead add a few teaspoons of either balsamic vinegar or apple cider vinegar with a little extra virgin olive oil to add some healthy fats. There's no need to put sugar on your next salad.

Refined White Carbohydrates

Just like refined sugar is striped of health benefits such as vitamins, nutrients and fiber, so are refined grains. By refined grains, I am referring to white bread, pasta, white rice, many breakfast cereals, bakery items such as cookies and cakes; heck, I'm pretty much referring to every pre-packaged snack food in the grocery store. They all contain enriched wheat flour. These refined grains might not be sugar, but they quickly digest into simple sugars, causing blood sugar levels to spike and then crash almost as quickly, leading to a crash in your energy level and to more cravings. Consuming these foods is very much the same as consuming refined sugar as far as your body is concerned, leading to such issues as weight gain, inflammation, type II diabetes and all of the other things we've discussed. It's just best to stay away from them. If you feel the urge to snack, have some nuts like almonds or walnuts, which will satisfy your appetite with good fats, fiber and protein. Or just prepare some healthy snack foods at home from scratch so you know exactly what you're eating. You can even just try drinking water. As I've said before, sometimes thirst just comes disguised as hunger.

Tomato Sauce

You may not have suspected this guy of containing the sweet white powder, but tomato sauce definitely does, wrecking havoc on the blood sugar levels in everyone. It doesn't matter if it is canned or jarred. This even includes ketchup. So the next time you buy tomato sauce, look for the label that says low sugar (make sure there are no artificial sweeteners). Or if you're so inclined, you can always make your own tomato sauce using fresh tomatoes and herbs, knowing that you'd never put sugar into it.

Low Fat Fruit Yogurt

Don't get me wrong, yogurt can be highly nutritious. There's just one problem. Not all yogurt is the same. Just like many low fat foods in general, low fat fruit yogurts have sugar added to them to enhance their flavor. Low fat fruit yogurt can have up to 40 grams of sugar and sometimes more, roughly the daily limit for an adult. **IN ONE CUP!** So if you love yogurt like I do, do yourself the favor of going with full fat, natural, or Greek yogurt, which has more health benefits and much less sugar. Avoid the yogurt sweetened by added sugar.

BBQ Sauce

BBQ sauce is sooo tasty as a marinade or dip. Wonder why? Well, two tablespoons of it contain approximately 14 grams of sugar. In fact, up to 40% of BBQ sauce may well be pure sugar! If you like to splatter your steak with it, you could be consuming large amounts of sugar without even meaning to. If you love your BBQ sauce, then always check the labels to choose the sauce with the least amount of sugar. And be very mindful of how much sauce you do use. Measure out what a serving size actually is.

Sports Drinks

These drinks have their purpose. They are formulated to hydrate and fuel highly trained athletes during prolonged and intense periods of physical training. That is why sports drinks are filled with high amounts of added sugars, which can be quickly absorbed by these athletes and then used for energy. Most of us do not fall into this category. We should just stick to water. In fact, for most of us, these are no better than the sugary drinks that were discussed earlier in this chapter. 32 grams of sugar in a standard 20 ounce bottle doesn't lie. Also note that vitamin water and flavored water fall into this category as well, with each having about the same amount of sugar as sports drinks. Better to just have an "all in one" vitamin with a glass of water. If you need to add some flavor to it, just add a piece of lemon (like I said before), which is always thirst quenching. Coconut water is another replacement option as it is thirst quenching and full of vitamins and nutrients, although it does contain some sugar, so be careful with it.

Granola

You might think of granola as a good low fat healthy snack. Granola bars too. Well, the main ingredient is oats, so that's a great start as oats contain the protein, fat and fiber that we're looking for. The only problem is that the oats are combined with honey and other added sweeteners such as brown sugar, which greatly increases the amount of sugar and calories that these oats contain. In fact, a one ounce granola bar contains eight grams of sugar. If you like granola, then it's best to add it as a topping on fruit or yogurt (not low fat) instead of filling an entire bowl with it.

Canned Fruit

All fruit contains natural sugars. And that is perfectly fine. However, there is a problem with canned fruit. Canned fruit is processed. Many times during this processing, the fruit is peeled and preserved in a sugary syrup, which unfortunately adds a lot of sugar to what many people view as a healthy snack. The canning process can also destroy vitamin C, although other nutrients tend to be well preserved. Always go for whole fruit, which has all of the health benefits that one would expect with less sugar. If you do want to eat canned fruit, go for the fruit preserved in fruit juice instead of syrup, which tends to have much less added sugar.

Flavored Coffees

These drinks are very popular nowadays. However, the amount of sugar hidden in them can blow your mind. A large flavored coffee from some chains can contain up to 100 grams of added sugar, the equivalent of 25 teaspoons. That is up to three times the amount of sugar you would find in a 12 ounce can of Coke. If you stop and think about the link between sugary drinks and poor health, then you know that it's best to stick with a standard coffee without any of the flavored syrups or added sugar. Also, some people, after quitting sugar, will even start to enjoy their coffee black again. This is due to the adjustment of the taste buds.

Iced Tea

As I'm sure you already know, iced tea is a tea that has been chilled. What you may not have known is that it is also sweetened with added sugar or flavored with syrup. The sugar content can vary. However, the ones that are commercially prepared contain approximately 33 grams of sugar per 12 ounce serving. That is about the same as a can of Coke. If you love your tea, go with the regular tea or pick one that doesn't have sugar added.

Protein Bars

This is a very popular snack and it's not hard to see why. It's marketed as very healthy and is full of protein. Protein will help you feel fuller with less food, leading to less calorie intake, thereby helping with weight loss. It also helps build and maintain muscle mass, something that is very important for our health. These factors have led the world to believe that protein bars are a healthy snack. However, many have added sugar that can make them less than healthy. Some may contain 30 grams of sugar, which approximates a candy bar. When choosing one, just read the label to avoid the ones high in sugar.

Jams, Preserves, and Spreads (Marmalade)

It's best to be careful if you like to put a little jelly on your toast. What you spread on your toast may be up to 60 percent pure sugar. There's no fat and very little in the way of fiber and protein. That won't help to satisfy your appetite and will lead to cravings. If you have to have any spreads, then use them sparingly.

Breakfast Cereals

Many are advertised as healthy, however, they tend to contain a lot of sugar. In fact, over 90 percent of cold cereals sold in the United States are preloaded with added sugars. The average cold cereal contains about nine grams of sugar per serving, which is much less than a bowl. Just measure out one serving. It's usually just one cup. And over 20 percent of the average cold cereal's weight is just pure sugar. Think about that before having a bowl of cereal for breakfast or feeding it to your kids. Some do come with a good amount of vitamins and minerals, but there's a way to get them without consuming so much sugar. Just find the cereal that has no added sugar or a low amount of added sugar such as Cheerios, Rice Krispies (gluten free) and Corn Flakes. Again, check the labels to find the low sugar cereals. And add your own touch to the low sugar cereal such as almonds and/or fruit such as blueberries or a chopped banana. This will help you feel fuller so your blood sugar levels can stay consistent throughout the day.

Instant Oatmeal

Most people know oatmeal to be healthy. However, some packaged varieties of instant oatmeal can contain up to 14 grams of sugar per packet. Instead, just add some nuts, fruits, and spices to the standard oatmeal. This will allow you to add flavor to it while reaping all of the health benefits that oatmeal has to offer. And without adding any refined sugar to boot.

Peanut Butter

Reading the label is very important when choosing peanut butter. Many brands, including Skippy and Jif, have around two teaspoons (eight grams) of sugar per serving. However, there are brands out there that have no added sugar including Trader Joe's and Smucker's Natural. The healthy peanut butter is worth finding.

Frozen Meals

These meals seem like a great idea when we're exhausted and just don't have the energy to cook or pick something up on the way home. So convenient they are. There is just one problem. Many contain anywhere from 20 to 40 grams of sugar, especially those covered in sauces or are low-fat (recurring theme). Again, labels tell all. Always read them before choosing a frozen dinner if you greatly value their convenience. In many cases, however, the extra sugar is not worth the convenience. An easy option in place of frozen meals is to just bake a fillet of chicken or fish in the oven with a fresh avocado and a fresh tomato as sides. Just slice the avocado and tomato into pieces and you have yourself a nice healthy meal that is so easy to make.

Smoothies

Fruit and veggie smoothies are a tasty, healthy drink, right? Well, not always. Although packed with fruits, vegetables, and other ingredients that benefit our health, smoothies are also another source of sugar. Many have sugar and sweeteners added to enhance their natural flavor. In fact, some smoothies can contain up to 60 to 70 grams of sugar. It's always best to check the nutritional facts online before visiting a smoothie franchise so that you can make the healthiest choice possible. Or you can just make them yourself at home. Then you can know for sure that no sugar has been added to it.

Fake Fats

Stay away from vegetable oils and margarines as they are highly refined, inflammatory, and most importantly, won't make you feel satisfied. It's a terrible substitute for fat. Again, eat the food with the healthy fats and your health will improve. Use butter instead of margarine. And instead of vegetable oil, there are much healthier choices, among them are olive oil, coconut oil, and avocado oil.

Worst Fruits (In terms of sugar content only)

Some fruits have higher sugar content compared to others. That is not to say that you should never eat these fruits but keep in mind that too many of them can elevate your blood sugar level. Of course they won't elevate your blood sugar levels to the point of the previous foods discussed. Like many things in life, moderation is key. Figs and grapes contain the most. Both contain 16 grams of sugar per 100 gram serving. Mangoes and pomegranates are next at 14 grams of sugar per 100 gram serving. Bananas have 12 grams per 100 gram serving. Cherries have 8 grams per 100 gram serving. Nothing wrong with having a banana or a few grapes, just watch how many you eat. Remember, all of these fruits have nutritional value as well.

Although this list is a great start to knowing what not to eat, keep in mind that it is not exhaustive. Just read and understand the labels. Don't assume anything about the sugar content of what you consume. And don't forget, low fat almost always means high sugar. Knowing what has sugar is half the battle. However, it means nothing if you don't fight by limiting your sugar intake. You can start fighting right away by replacing the above foods with foods that don't have added sugar, which leads us to the next chapter.

Chapter 6

What Should I Add To My Diet?

In the quest to end sugar's control over your diet, there are certain foods that should absolutely be added. Remember that what you eat is everything in ending your sugar dependence and in maintaining a healthy low sugar diet once sugar's control over you has ended. You want to eat foods that include fiber, protein and healthy fats. I know I keep repeating that but it's so important to remember. The healthiest foods are the most nutritionally dense foods found in their original forms. Keep in mind that you want to limit fruit to about two servings per day if you've just started the detox process. There are some camps that advise not to eat any fruit whatsoever during that time. It's entirely up to you which route you want to take (although the withdrawals will be more difficult to handle if you completely ban fruit). It's also a good idea to add foods that are naturally sweet without sugar, such as cinnamon and vanilla extract. You don't have to eat every healthy food on this list but try different things to see what you like and what you don't like. It's also a good idea to prepare these foods in different ways (without adding sugar or other unhealthy things of course). Here are some foods that are absolutely worth adding to your diet:

Almonds

These nuts contain lots of healthy fats, protein, fiber, magnesium and vitamin E. Their consumption helps lower blood sugar levels. Almonds also reduces hunger. Just a small amount, like a handful a day, can deliver these terrific benefits. Just mix them in a salad or a low sugar cereal like Cheerios.

Apples

Containing twice the fiber of other common fruits like peaches and grapes while containing antioxidants as well, apples definitely do their part to maintain your blood sugar level and prevent cravings. They have most definitely earned the phrase, "an apple a day keeps the doctor away" and is good to have handy as a snack.

Avocado

"An avocado a day will keep the doctor away" definitely works as a true statement as well. These fruits are tremendously nutritious. In fact, some call it a perfect food. They contain fiber and healthy fats as well as high levels of vitamin C, vitamin E and potassium (more than bananas). The fiber content helps maintain blood sugar levels, important to stopping those cravings. The healthy fats in avocados also help improve insulin function.

Bananas

Bananas are one of the most nutritionally dense foods that are found in nature. If there's one down side, it's that there is a decent amount of sugar in them relative to their fiber content compared to other fruits like apples or blueberries. Just watch how many you eat if you are just starting to quit sugar. Otherwise I wouldn't worry too much about them. Their nutritional value far outweighs the negative effects of their sugar content. Add them to a sugar-free cereal in the morning.

Blueberries

One of the healthiest foods around, blueberries are considered by many a superfood. It is high in fiber and water content. It has a low glycemic index, which means that it digests more slowly, delaying hunger cues and helping to better control your appetite. This means less cravings. And that is just the start. It is also full of antioxidants and vitamins. You can't go wrong with them and you can reap their health benefits with just a couple of handfuls per day. Just like bananas and almonds, they are a nice addition to a sugar-free cereal.

Chia Seeds

Among the most nutrient dense foods that you'll find, chia seeds are full of fiber, proteins, and omega-3 fats. In fact, a single ounce of them contains eleven grams of fiber, four grams of protein and five grams of omega-3 fats. Chia seeds in general contain a large percentage of the recommended intake for many nutrients. They can even improve athletic performance on par with a sports drink without the sugar, although that claim is only based on limited studies. No wonder these wondrous seeds were so revered by the Maya and the Aztecs! It's a nice addition to standard oatmeal.

Chicken Breast

High in protein yet low in calories, this well known staple is great to put on the dinner plate. Chicken breast is also full of many nutrients. Baking is the healthiest way to prepare it. Avoid frying chicken breast as it will add unhealthy fats.

Cinnamon

This is a spice that is rather sweet without sugar. That sweet taste can help calm a craving. It may even lower, yes lower, blood sugar levels. It does so by forcing the muscle cells to remove sugar from the bloodstream, where it is converted into energy. Cinnamon also increases sensitivity to insulin, leading to better blood sugar control overall. Sprinkle it on different foods as a sugar substitute whenever you get that sugar craving. Its sweetness may be all that you need to get through it.

Coconut Oil

Coconut oil is great for dealing with sugar cravings as it is slightly sweet in flavor while containing healthy fats. You can cook or bake it into your food to prevent yourself from feeling deprived of sugar. Also, if you like sugar in your coffee, try blending coconut oil into it instead for a rich tasting energy boost. There is a need to take care with the amount you use as it is high in fat and can easily lead to weight gain.

Coconut Water

Coconut water is a great replacement for soda or a sports drink. This stuff satisfies the sweet tooth while containing much lower sugar than soda and fruit juices at about 9.1 grams in a 12 ounce drink, compared to a 12 ounce can of soda, which can contain up to 40 grams of sugar. And it's full of potassium and even has some protein. Have it straight out of the coconut when on a tropical vacation or have one of the packaged varieties (just read the label to make sure nothing is added to it). Don't overindulge in the coconut water, however, as like a juice or soda, it's easy to consume too much as there is no fiber to make you feel full. I also wouldn't drink it during the initial quitting period. After that quitting period, a few a week probably won't hurt you.

Eggs

Eggs are super-nutritious as they contain all of the nutrients required to turn a single cell into a baby chicken. Each egg has six grams of protein and five grams of healthy fats, all coming from just under 80 calories. They are also extremely fulfilling. Eating them at breakfast will make it easier to say no to sugar all day long. Not a bad idea to replace that bagel in the morning with an egg instead, huh? The easiest way to prepare them is to hard boil them.

Flaxseeds

Flaxseeds have been used for centuries for medicinal and health purposes. In fact, they can be used to reduce inflammation. They provide protein, healthy fats, and are high in fiber. Flaxseeds are also full of minerals like magnesium, potassium, and zinc. Sprinkle them in salads and standard oatmeal.

Kale

This green is more nutritious than the rest. It is a terrific source of calcium, fiber, vitamin C, iron and many other vitamins. It also has more antioxidants than most other fruits and vegetables and are loaded with compounds that are believed to fight cancer. It even contains protein. And to top it all off, it is very low in calories with just 33 calories in a single cup raw. In fact, it is one of the most nutritionally dense foods that exist today. It can be prepared in many different ways from boiled or steamed to roasted. You can even eat it as a chip! Oh yeah, and it's low in sugar. However you add kale to your diet, it is well worth the effort.

Lentils

High in protein and essential nutrients while being cheap and easy to prepare, lentils are a great addition to your diet. They help to maintain blood sugar levels as they are low on the glycemic index.

Oatmeal

A whole-grain powerhouse that stands the test of time by providing great nutrition. Keep in mind that I am not referring to instant oatmeal, which can contain a fair amount of sugar, as I mentioned in the previous chapter. Oatmeal is full of, you guessed it, oats, which contain a ton of satisfying, soluble fiber. You can even add more nutrition and flavor by throwing some flaxseed or walnuts onto it as well as other things. Or if you want to add some sweetness without adding refined sugar, try some cinnamon and/or fruit? There are so many ways that you can make oatmeal a great start to the day!

Quinoa

This small, grain-like seed packs a huge nutritional punch. So nutritious, in fact, that it was revered by the Inca, who believed it to be sacred. It's high in fiber and protein, with nine essential amino acids. In fact, a cup of cooked quinoa contains eight grams of protein and five grams of fiber. It even contains a small amount of omega-3 fatty acids. There are three main types: red, white and black. It's a great substitute for rice.

Salmon

This fish is a great addition to your diet. High in protein, omega-3 fatty acids, and vitamin D, it's one of the healthiest things that you can put on your plate. Look for wild salmon, as farmed salmon tends to contain several times more toxins, although their levels are still far less than what is considered dangerous and would be more than offset by this fish's nutritional bounty.

Sauerkraut

There is some bacteria in your gut that thrives on sugar, which increases your sugar cravings. Sauerkraut, as a fermented vegetable, can help bring your gut bacteria into balance, which helps in decreasing the power of those cravings.

Sweet Potatoes

The word "sweet" may be in the name, but don't keep them out of your sugar-free diet. They are full of fiber and potassium. Their sweetness helps with managing cravings. And if you want to make your sweet potatoes even sweeter, just sprinkle a little cinnamon onto them.

Walnuts

An excellent source of healthy fats, including omega-3, as well as protein and fiber, walnuts are quite the nutritional snack. They even contain antioxidants and cancer fighting properties. In fact, the dietary fat found in walnuts have been found in studies to reduce fasting insulin levels in overweight adults with type 2 diabetes. It's not a stretch to believe that they can help other people in the same way.

This is not an exhaustive list, just like the previous chapter. But it's a great start! As always, whole fruit and vegetables, lean meats, nuts and seeds and anything else that is not processed will be your best friend in your fight against sugar. Always have that on your mind when you're shopping at the grocery store. That is the biggest key.

Chapter 7

Can I still have fun after starting my new sugar-free life?

Sometimes we still want to enjoy the sweeter things. And really, that's fine. What's the point of life if you can't enjoy it? If you're so strict that you feel like you can't have anything that you love, then you may end up feeling miserable. This feeling makes life more difficult in general. It can even interfere with socializing as it seems everybody else can eat what they want and you find yourself envious. They sometimes even point it out which can make things feel awkward. I'm here to say not to worry. Have something once in a while. It's fine. Just keep in mind that it's not a good idea to consume anything with added sugar if you are still in the initial quitting period (first two weeks). This is especially true with alcohol, as it taxes your liver beyond what is done to it by the sugar detoxing itself. However, once you make it past that point, you might want to return a little back to normal. And by normal, I don't mean reverting back to your old ways but just to be mindful of your choices. Beyond that, there are still some nice options when you eat out. The restaurant menu isn't always going to have all of the information that you need to make the most informed decision, but there are some things that can be done to help you make good choices. Let's go over some of them.

An important one is to be prepared. If you know which restaurant you are going to eat at ahead of time, look up the menu online. And if you are not sure which plate is a good sugar-free option, then go ahead and call the restaurant. Let them know what you are looking for. Most of them will be happy to answer any question that you have and will make any necessary adjustments. Remember, restaurants are a business and businesses want their customers to be happy. They also want you to come back. It's how they stay profitable.

Once you have a good idea of what is on the menu, have a healthy sugar-free snack before you leave for the restaurant. This will help prevent you from eating the entire breadbasket and any other high carb appetizer. And drink water only. No juices. No sodas. If you have to drink coffee, then stay black or choose a flat white. Milk-based coffees tend to have a lot of sugar.

As you are looking through the menu for your meal (either online or at the restaurant), look out for clues that can indicate sugar. Any ingredient or description that indicates sweetness has to be considered sugar. Examples include glazed, balsamic, caramelized and even the word sweet itself. If you choose a steak, chicken breast or fish as the main dish, you're doing well, as long as they are not fried or battered. A large salad is good too. However, once you get to the sauces and dressings, things can easily start going wrong. Many tomato sauces, barbeque sauces and salad dressings are high in sugar. If you really want to have a sauce or dressing, it's better to have it on the side so that you can better control how much you consume. Better yet, ask about their sugar content. If your server can't tell you, ask what brand it is and look it up on your smartphone. Ask the server to tell you all of the sauces that are available. Sometimes the best option is to just ditch the sauces and to stick to salt, pepper, and olive oil. In fact, as a salad dressing, olive oil is the best as it has no sugar and is full of healthy fats. Also try mustards, gravies and homemade mayonnaise as they are good choices for other dishes. Smart substitutions for side dishes and appetizers are very important. Choose veggies, salads, fruit and whole grains like quinoa in place of white bread, white rice, french fries and pasta as the later group is quickly converted into glucose by your body, raising blood sugar levels. If you almost always opt for foods that contain plenty of fiber, protein and healthy fats, then you'll always be fine.

While having that nice meal with friends, it'd be nice to have a drink too, right? There's nothing wrong with a couple (as in one or two a couple times a month) of drinks once in a while. Keep in mind that this advice is only for people who haven't had alcohol problems. Otherwise, it's good to enjoy life while keeping things in moderation. And although alcoholic drinks generally aren't the healthiest, there are three that tend to be better than the rest when it comes to sugar: beer, wine and dry spirits.

Beer does have a lot of sugar, but not in the form of fructose, which is the type of sugar that most easily converts to fat. Once you are beyond the initial quitting period, it is ok to drink beer in moderation, which is about a bottle a day or less. Maybe have one with your dinner after a hard day. In fact, there are even some studies that suggest that a 12 ounce bottle of beer a day can have a beneficial effect on your health, although the jury is still out on that.

Wine is something I'm sure most of us would like to have with a meal as well. And that's perfectly fine. A five ounce glass of red wine contains less than a gram of sugar. Dry white wines like Chardonnay are also low in sugar and are a good choice. Again, moderation is key. With that being said, there are some studies suggesting that drinking a glass of red wine (again, five ounces) a day can have many health benefits. Who am I to dispute scientific studies? If you can stick to just one five ounce glass a day, then why not?

Want something stronger? Dry spirits are very low in fructose and are also fine in moderation. These include whiskey, gin, and vodka. Again, always in moderation. If you don't want to drink them straight, just mix them with soda water and a lime.

Remember that not all drinks are created equal when it comes to sugar. Avoid dessert wines, ciders, liqueurs and cocktails when getting your drink on, as almost all will contain a ton of sugar.

There is one more thing to note. Although it's fine to drink alcohol in moderation, it is an addictive substance that comes with its own baggage of health problems. If you've had an addiction with alcohol in the past, it's best to stay away from it altogether. Also understand that alcohol, if you drink too much, can lead to bad decision making, which often include decisions regarding your diet. You are more likely to grab that piece of cake while under the influence. And not only cake, but a whole lot of other not so healthy food too. It's always something worth considering.

Besides alcohol, you may want to have sweets once in a while too. I know. I know. I said keep things like cake, candy, and bakery items out of your diet. Whether or not you want to reintroduce any of these things into your life a few weeks or months after quitting is up to you. If you don't feel comfortable eating any of these things, then don't. If you don't feel like you have the discipline to stop yourself if you do have any sweets, then again, don't. Otherwise, a piece of cake at a birthday party or a piece of candy every once in a while won't hurt. I would limit it to maybe a couple of times a week, maybe less. Don't allow yourself to get into the habit of consistently eating these things as that's where you'll ultimately hurt yourself.

One thing that is both sweet and healthy is dark chocolate. Not to be confused with milk chocolate, which has little nutritional value, dark chocolate, or chocolate that is at least 70% cacao has several health benefits and is an excellent substitute for any chocolate in general. It contains fiber, has plenty of vitamins and minerals, and is a terrific source of antioxidants. Some studies even show that it can improve cardiovascular health. It still has some sugar so eat it in moderation. One to two servings a day (but don't eat it at all during the initial quitting period) is probably fine. I wouldn't eat any more than that however.

Treating yourself is such a wonderful thing. It's one of the great small pleasures of life. However, if you're going to treat yourself, always make sure that you do it with something that you absolutely love. For example, if you like donuts alright, but don't particularly love them, don't eat them. If you are going to eat something that is unhealthy, make sure that it is something that you love, otherwise, it won't be worth it. Always consider how much you enjoy something in comparison to how healthy that something is before consuming it. And if you do overindulge, don't sweat it. Just get back on the right path and forget about your mistake. It happens. We all make them. One bad day won't ruin your new lifestyle unless you let it. If you follow that up with 10, 100 or 1000 days where you do the right thing, that bad day won't even register.

Another thing to keep in mind. Never focus on what you

can't eat. Instead, focus on the great variety of available foods that you CAN eat. If you do that, you will be less likely to feel deprived. You will feel more satisfied. And of course, you will be happier. Always focus on improving your health and all of the new things that it will allow you to do in your life.

Chapter 8

What are other names for sugar?

It is a difficult thing to determine how much added sugar is in a food product as added sugar has so many names. Even after accounting for all of the different names, how do you judge how much of a particular food product is made from added sugar relative to other ingredients? Well, as I said in **Chapter 2**, the ingredients are listed in descending order according to their weight. In other words, food products that list a sugar source at or near the top/beginning of the ingredient list or have more than one sugar source overall can be counted on to have a large amount of refined sugar. Here are the most common names for sugar that you may see on the labels:

- agave nectar
- beet sugar
- brown sugar
- cane crystals
- cane juice
- cane sugar
- caramel
- corn sweetener
- corn syrup
- crystalline fructose
- dextran
- dextrose
- evaporated cane juice
- fructose
- fruit juice concentrates
- glucose
- high-fructose corn syrup
- honey
- inver sugar
- maltose

- malt syrup
- maple syrup
- molasses
- raw sugar
- sucrose
- syrup

This isn't an exhaustive list as I just wanted to list the most common sugar synonyms that are used. If a word has sugar, syrup, juice, or has **-ose** in the name, then you can count on that word being another name for sugar. If you aren't sure about an ingredient, just research it. We all have smartphones. The ability to look anything up is right in your pocket.

To Conclude

Quitting added sugar is a huge decision that will have huge ramifications. It is something that can be very difficult in the beginning but once you get through it, you will find yourself living a higher quality of life.

You will have broken away from the addiction that was slowly poisoning you, possibly to an early grave. After giving up sugar, you will feel and look better. You will feel and look younger. You will start to be able to do things that you haven't been able to do since your younger days and possibly do things you haven't ever been able to do before.

It only takes a few things to move forward. The most important thing is having the right mindset. Without that, the rest doesn't really matter. You need to make all the small decisions with one goal in mind. The positive effects of these decisions will then compound into huge positive results in the long run. After getting your mind right, learn how to read the labels Also learn how much actual food is in a serving size. Measure out what a serving size actually is for each food product. That is the only way to fully understand what is actually in your food. Then replace the processed foods in your diet with healthy whole foods. Stay in the produce, meat and dairy sections of the supermarket as much as possible to find those healthy whole foods. Stay away from the middle aisles. That is where all of the processed foods with the refined sugar is found. Another important point, just drink plain old water when thirsty. No more juices, sodas, energy drinks, etc. And when the cravings and withdrawals come, handle them as best as you can. Use natural sweeteners like cinnamon or have a piece of fruit if that helps. Also participate in productive activities that help keep your mind off of those withdrawals, such as sewing or biking. This will also keep you from transferring the addiction of sugar to another negative addiction such as gambling or excessive shopping. And lastly, if you fail, it's only temporary. Just forget it and go back to the positive things that you were doing before. Just keep going. We all fail at things that are hard to do. There's no shame in it. Just don't quit. One bad decision won't undue all of your hard work. If the vast majority of your little decisions bring you closer to your goal, there's no need to sweat. Just keep your eye on the prize; the prize of a longer, higher quality of life.

Once you reach this newfound higher quality of life, it will lead you to a new place where you will be more likely to find contentment. And that is the most important thing, as happiness is everything. You'll find yourself sick less often, while having more energy, with fewer worries overall. You'll find yourself wanting to do more, like spend more time playing with your kids and grandkids. Or maybe try some exciting new hobbies like hiking or swimming. A new adventure will await you.

So what are you waiting for? Tomorrow won't be any better if you don't change what you do today first.

Now let's get started!!!

I would like to thank you for purchasing my book. I hope you've enjoyed it. I know that if you apply what you've learned in this book that you can take your health to heights. If you have enjoyed this book and found its information helpful, please leave a review. I would so greatly appreciate it. If you have any questions, please contact me at jjkozpublishing@gmail.com. Good luck on your journey to a healthier life. And again, I can't thank you enough that you chose my book. Thank you!

9 781976 216749